DEDICATION

I dedicate this book to my wife who is always there at my worst and keeps on motivating me to be at my best. I also dedicate this book to everybody who has lost hope in getting that healthy lifestyle. May this book serve as an inspiration to you all.

TABLE OF CONTENTS

7 Habits of Healthy People: The Simple Guide

Helpful Tips of Healthy People

By: Walter Gregory

9781634289887

PUBLISHERS NOTES

Disclaimer – Speedy Publishing LLC

This publication is intended to provide helpful and informative material. It is not intended to diagnose, treat, cure, or prevent any health problem or condition, nor is intended to replace the advice of a physician. No action should be taken solely on the contents of this book. Always consult your physician or qualified health-care professional on any matters regarding your health and before adopting any suggestions in this book or drawing inferences from it.

The author and publisher specifically disclaim all responsibility for any liability, loss or risk, personal or otherwise, which is incurred as a consequence, directly or indirectly, from the use or application of any contents of this book.

Any and all product names referenced within this book are the trademarks of their respective owners. None of these owners have sponsored, authorized, endorsed, or approved this book.

Always read all information provided by the manufacturers' product labels before using their products. The author and publisher are not responsible for claims made by manufacturers.

This book was originally printed before 2014. This is an adapted reprint by Speedy Publishing LLC with newly updated content designed to help readers with much more accurate and timely information and data.

Speedy Publishing LLC

40 E Main Street,Newark,Delaware,19711

Contact Us: 1-888-248-4521

Website: http://www.speedypublishing.co

REPRINTED Paperback Edition: ISBN: 9781634289887

Manufactured in the United States of America

Chapter 1- Overview to 7 Habits of Healthy People

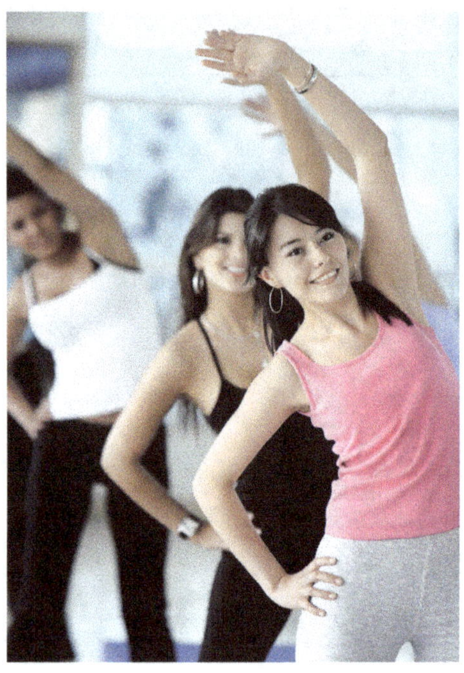

If certain experts are to be believed, we are currently facing a crisis the likes of which we have never seen before; we are being faced with a global obesity epidemic.

Since 1980, the number of people suffering from obesity has literally more than doubled, with there being 1.4 billion overweight adults, and 500 million who can be considered as obese.

As far as children go, the numbers just keep on climbing, with certain countries seeing more than a quarter of their kids suffering from obesity. Long story short, if things keep on going the way they do, then in a few decades most of the world's population will be obese, if of course we even manage to survive that long. In order to fight this great plague it is important what it stems from… just like with any huge problem, there are numerous causes in play here.

For starters, we are leading increasingly sedentary lifestyles. Long gone are the days when we ploughed fields twelve hours a day or dug up coal in mines... long gone are the days when most people had to dedicate their working time to physical labor. These days, most people work sitting, or perhaps standing still, and needless to say, there isn't much effort involved in that, at least in a physical sense. The problem however is that even though we reduced our level of activity we kept on increasing how much we ate. As a result, our bodies simply aren't subjected to enough exercise to burn all the excess calories we gain, which leads to a noticeable weight gain. However, a lack of exercising coupled with overeating is not the only source of this problem.

Another cause for what we are observing today can be traced to economic fluctuations in regards to food prices. As it happens, in most cases, the cheaper a food is, the more filling and unhealthy it is. More specifically, the fast food industry is being referenced. Junk food restaurants have established themselves in countless poorer countries and economically-disadvantaged areas, providing people with cheap and fattening alternatives that allow them to save money. What's more, these alternatives are sometimes even tastier. In the end, the point is that the cost of healthy foods exceeds that of unhealthy ones.

Understanding proper diet can aid you in bodybuilding. Many people make the mistake of thinking that all foods containing fat are bad for your body when bodybuilding. The real truth is that a proper balance of fat and other food groups can accelerate your physical development. It can also be underestimated concerning how important protein is to the bodybuilder. On average a bodybuilder should consume 1.2 g of protein per lb. of bodyweight. Protein is not the only important nutritional component of bodybuilding, achieving the adequate ratio of carbohydrate to protein consumption is also important.

Steroids are not the only way to get the body desired by bodybuilders. Those professionals who value being healthy will tell you that good training principals include the understanding that you need to combine a nutrient-rich diet with the proper amount of rest. This proper combo will give you the edge you need to create the body that family and friends will envy.

It is also a misconception that those who start bodybuilding may have and that is that they should work faster or do more reps to build muscle. The truth is that you need to rest and workout for best results. A good schedule is to alternate workout days with rest days. Another good idea is to build your rep sequence by 5. This workout/rest and rep build up by 5 is a good combination to keep in mind to build muscle mass.

Many beginners to bodybuilding will make the mistake of thinking that more reps you complete or the more equipment time or dumbbell time you log in, the faster you build muscle. A principal of bodybuilding is that it is important to work out until the muscle is fatigued. Each set is different and depending on what exercise you are doing, you may actually fatigue out muscle fibers in one set. You should concentrate on creating the kind of intensity in your workout that will allow you to drop or break-down sets so that you can actually rep out, by lowering the weight and then continue reps until you either cannot complete another rep or you run out of weight.

When you know the true facts about bodybuilding you can use them in your workout plan to give you a healthier and more productive workout. You can train your mind to follow the truth about bodybuilding much like you can have the discipline regarding the training of your body. Discipline on two levels - body and mind.

Now with what we've just covered and as we begin this guide, it's important to realize that the world is in a bad state, health wise. But you don't have to accept what is happening in society. You are about to learn the 7 keys to transform your body and quite literally it will transform your life! So dive in, read, absorb and put into practice exactly what you learn here and see the change happen. You have the power in your hands to change your health and live the life you want to, rest assured that in the end, your body will thank you for it.

Chapter 2- Key Habit 1 – Breakfast is a Must!

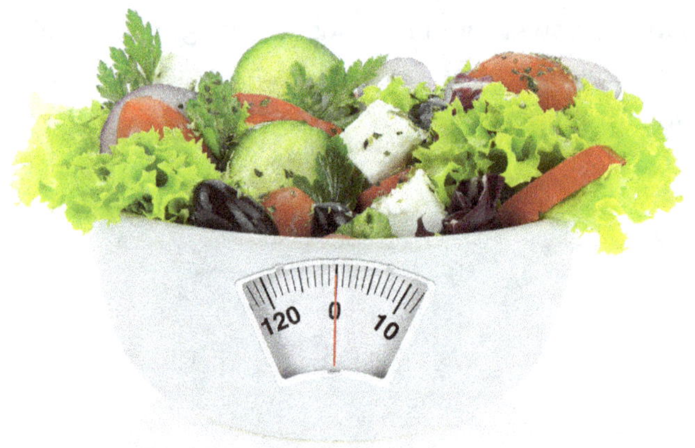

If certain experts are to be believed, we are currently facing a crisis the likes of which we have never seen before; we are being faced with a global obesity epidemic.

Since 1980, the number of people suffering from obesity has literally more than doubled, with there being 1.4 billion overweight adults, and 500 million who can be considered as obese.

As far as children go, the numbers just keep on climbing, with certain countries seeing more than a quarter of their kids suffering from obesity. Long story short, if things keep on going the way they do, then in a few decades most of the world's population will be obese, if of course we even manage to survive that long. In order to fight this great plague it is important what it stems from... just like with any huge problem, there are numerous causes in play here.

For starters, we are leading increasingly sedentary lifestyles. Long gone are the days when we ploughed fields twelve hours a day or dug up coal in mines... long gone are the days when most people had to dedicate their working time to physical labor. These days, most people work sitting, or perhaps standing still, and needless to say, there isn't much effort involved in that, at least in a physical sense. The problem however is that even though we reduced our level of activity we kept on increasing how much we ate. As a result, our bodies simply aren't subjected to enough exercise to burn all the excess calories we gain, which leads to a noticeable weight gain. However, a lack of exercising coupled with overeating is not the only source of this problem.

When losing weight, most individuals would skip eating breakfast thinking that it is an effective method of eliminating weight. Now, what they do not realize is that this technique is not really effective and could even cause negative effects on their bodies. When dieting, one of the most important things to be aware of is the importance of eating breakfast.

Breakfast is referred to "breakfast" simply because it breaks the long fast. People are asleep during the night for many hours, so in the morning, it is necessary to eat something in order to feel better and have the energy to face the new day. More importantly, having breakfast is vital to a fat burning diet. If you want to lose weight fast, be mindful to eat breakfast every day.

Here are some of the reasons and importance of eating breakfast to the body when dieting:

• Breakfast will allow you to control your hunger and avoid eating snacks later on during the day. What would be the use of your diet when you would eventually eat more because you are hungry, since you skipped breakfast? If ever you skipped breakfast, just ensure to have a healthy snack so that you can still lose weight effectively.

• A healthy breakfast will aid in increasing your body's metabolism-Eating breakfast can actually boost one's metabolism. If you skip breakfast, you would tend to place your body into starvation mode and try to conserve energy that it can. Now, when you eat breakfast, you are also telling your body that you are awake and you are not fasting anymore. This means that your body is ready to burn fat and utilizes the energy during the day.

• A healthy breakfast would also help you consume enough calories- Having enough calories is essential because this is responsible in increasing your energy levels. When you regularly skip breakfast, you are also not consuming calories that would end up in dropping off of your energy levels. This would also slow down your metabolism. Losing weight would be that effective.

• Eating breakfast is essential in losing weight, as it helps the body attain its weight loss goal faster. According to research and studies, those individuals who miss breakfast are the ones who were 4 times more likely to be overweight. If you do not want to risk of gaining weight, ensure not to skip breakfast.

These are some of the importance of eating breakfast to the body when dieting. Breakfast is the most essential meal of the day; therefore, it is necessary not to skip it. Of course, when dieting, just make sure that you follow a healthy breakfast so that you can efficiently lose weight and achieve your weight loss goals.

Eating breakfast is good and healthy, so do not think that skipping breakfast would help you lose weight. This will just make you feel weak and unhealthy, and this will not do well with your goal of losing weight. Have a healthy breakfast every day and follow the right diet. In no time, you would be surprised to see the positive results with your health and body.

Chapter 3- Key Habit 2 – Keep Hydrated

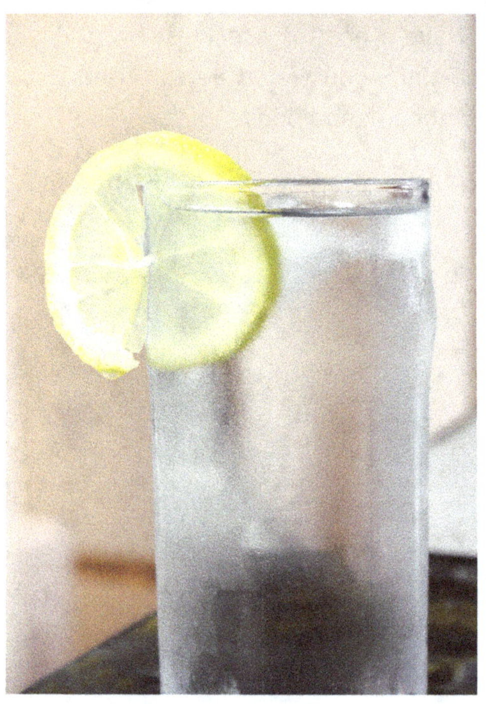

Drinking water plays a key role in dieting. If you ever find yourself stuck in a weight loss plateau despite following your diet program strictly, then it could be that you are not drinking enough water. Studies have shown that a lot people unsuspectingly suffer from severe or mild dehydration and you could be affected as well.

Your body requires water for various biochemical processes. The following are the benefits of drinking enough water to your body when dieting:

Water assists the body in the conversion of fat reserves into energy. When the body is dehydrated, the body's metabolism processes are slowed down and this impedes the breakdown of fats in the body, and in effect, your weight loss. If this happens, your weight loss curve hits a plateau.

Water holds naturally holds back your appetite. The hypothalamus region in your brain serves the role of controlling cravings and appetites, with the control centers for thirst and hunger situated next to one another. This means that drinking enough not only quenches your thirst, but it takes away the feelings of hunger as well. A study by Washington University found that drinking a glass of water before going to bed reduces mid-night cravings.

Water also helps in the prevention of sagging skin which is a common side effect of weight loss. It gives the skin a healthier and youthful look by helping in the reconstruction of destroyed skin cells.

Water assists in the elimination of waste products from the body. When dieting, the body loses weight and there are extra by products to be removed. This means that the body requires sufficient amounts of water into which the unwanted products will be dissolved and excreted from the body.

Water is effective in dealing with constipation. If the body does not get enough water, it is compelled to siphon it from its internal reserves, normally the colon, resulting into constipation. Normal bowel function will resume once the body receives adequate water.

In general, mild dehydration leads to a number of health complications. Mild dehydration is characterized by the following symptoms: fatigue, cravings, headaches and constipation. However, as soon as you get the water in balance, you achieve what diet experts refer to as a breakthrough point. At this point, as fluid retention in the body eases, the liver and endocrine systems start to operate more effectively, helping to reinstate your natural thirst, while reducing your cravings significantly. This eventually results into heightened metabolism rates which facilitate the breakdown and loss of fat in the body.

How Much Water Does the Body Need

In conclusion, the above benefits clearly show the importance of drinking water, particularly if you are on a diet. Nonetheless, everyone should make drinking water a habit. It should not only be done when you are thirsty as thirst, in itself, is an indication of the presence of dehydration. Hence, every adult ought to take at least eight glasses of water every day during cold weather. Since there is a lot of perspiration and loss of liquid during hot weather, additional glasses of water must be taken. Lastly, if exercises are part of your dieting plan, ensure that you drink 6-12 ounces of fluids after 15-20 intervals. This way, you will maintain the most favorable fluid balance during your exercises.

Chapter 4- Key Habit 4 – Sleep and Recovery

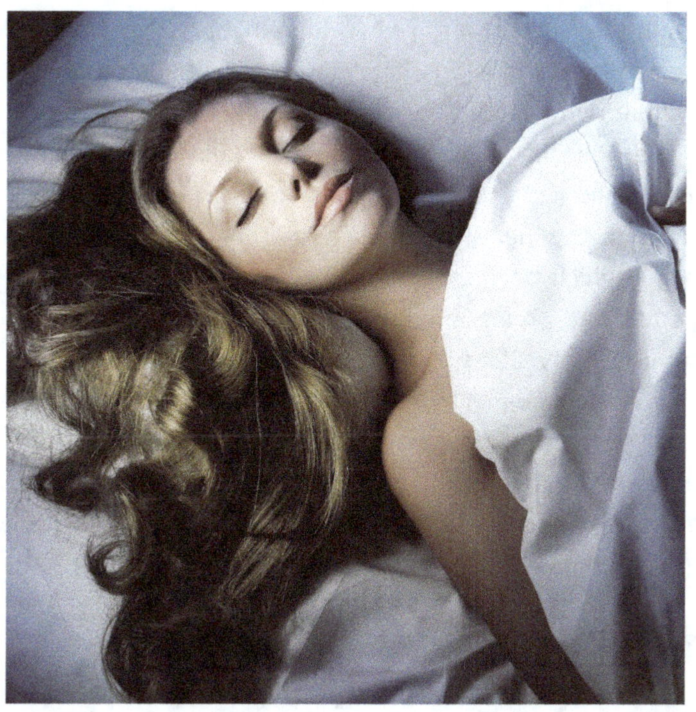

To consider sleep as an activity is difficult. One assumes sleep to be a phase of inactivity or rest. But, the matter of fact is, that sleep is that active phase in our entire day's routine, when numerous bodily functions are expedited. The sales data of sleep inducing tranquilizers and sleeping pills prove the rising cases of sleep deficiency that owes a lot to the modern lifestyle. While profound research is available on the importance of exercise for the body, few embark on the desire to learn about rest and sleep...yet it is one of the most important factors in overall health and well-being.

What Is Sleep?

Firstly, it's important to understand that while the body rests , the mind and the brain go on a restorative hyper-drive. Bodily signals are sent to the various organs of to begin its build up for the next hour of optimum action. The more sleep deprived a person is, the more the chances of deficient physical and mental activity, as you've not allowed your body to recover from the previous bout or prepare for the next. Sleep is a period of nerve and muscle relaxation which begins a period of repair and rejuvenation of all the tissues and organs, much needed after a day of hectic often strenuous activity. Sleep is determined by a certain biological cycle called as the 'circadian clock'. It depends on the intervals of certain number of hours of being awake followed by sleep, and so on. Other elements affecting it could be- the amount of light, stress levels, metabolism levels and even the medication we may be taking.

The Power of Sleep

Sleep is a powerful energy booster owing to the fact that while we sleep the process called 'anabolism' gets underway; understood more simply as the recovery process for cells and tissues through the production of enzymes and proteins. It in fact counteracts the effect of 'catabolism' or the process that occurs as you exercise or work- out during the day which produces an action wherein energy is released from cells. This affects the molecular components of the body. If your catabolism exceeds anabolism, little growth will happen. Thus those who strain themselves with a tougher workout or play an extra hour must give their body the extra rest to sustain their growth of muscle mass, which is directly proportionate to fitness.

There is no contention to the fact that mental alertness, concentration levels, communication, creativity, emotional balance and the productivity levels of an individual is also affected by the amount of sleep.

The Recovery Process

Prolonged sleep deprivation has been linked to anxiety and depression. Sleep induces the release of certain hormones that affect the central nervous system of the body thus affecting mood and emotional stability. Less sleep increases Cortisol which is a catabolic hormone and it decreases testosterone levels that are directly related to muscle mass gain. Less sleep also means a higher insulin level that increases your body's resistance to nutritional absorption.

While one can not contest the importance of fitness training including weight training one must understand the mechanics of what really happens to the body while this physical stress is being faced. While we exercise or lift weights, the muscle contracts or crunches thereby getting compressed or shortened.

This happens when the muscle microfibers compress. With every stimulus you give to your body, the muscle is strained to respond. What must however be realized is that between the phases of stimulus, the muscle needs to recover from it by building new bridges across the new muscle groups that are slowly forming. This growth is only possible when the body rests.

Another disturbing consequence that comes with compromising on the amount of sleep has is in the raised levels of cortisone which has been directly linked to more abdominal fats .While there has been encyclopedic quantum of research on the benefits of fitness programs, very little attention is paid to the importance of the body and its sleep requirement.

Balancing heavy workouts with its milder versions and adequate breaks from strenuous routines is not only the best antidote for perfect health; it's the best way to gain optimal benefits from your exercise routine.

Chapter 5- Key Habit 4 – Intense Cardio Training

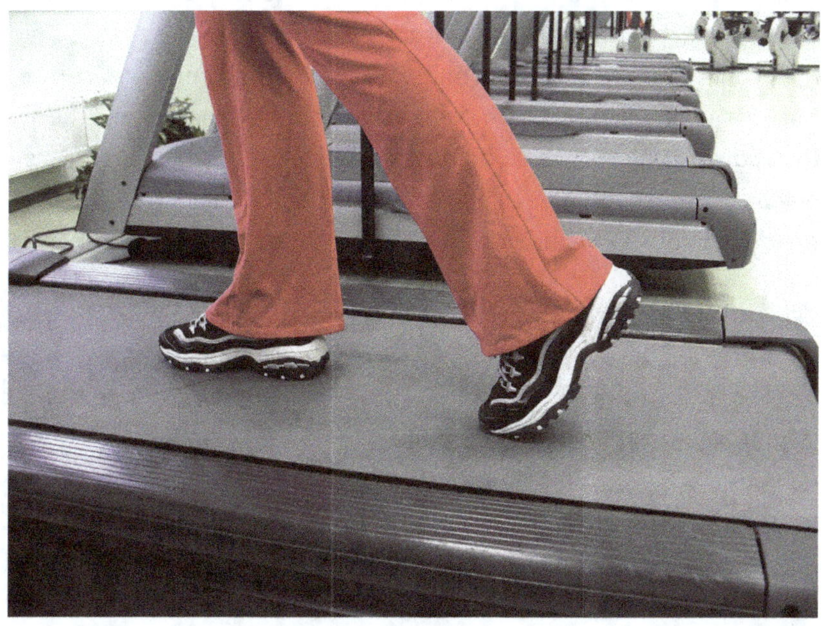

Using high intensity cardio to burn fat faster is an approach that has been used by a number of people, its benefits are huge and numerous, but it should always be done in a controlled environment and via a well set out plan. There is no doubt that this particular type of exercise does indeed burn fat a lot faster, but how does it actually work?

The reason why it works is because your body is being asked to produce a lot more energy than it has stored in order to deal with the intensity of the workout and it does this by burning off those fat reserves it has been keeping for a rainy day. Your body then has to keep producing energy even after you stop as it needs that in order to start repairing the muscles and settling your body after your strenuous workout.

It is also important to point out that this particular type of workout focuses on burning a different type of fat than what you would get doing a cardio workout that has a lower intensity such as a brisk walk. The problem with lower intensity cardio work is that it only gets your heart working to around 60% of the maximum heart rate, but this is not high enough for optimal fat burning in your body. Instead, you will only burn off the easy stuff, but the harder fat will still be there, so by increasing the intensity you burn off both types resulting in quicker weight loss.

There are other reasons why you should look at using this approach and one major reason is that you will then be able to deal with lactic acid a lot easier. It is this lactic acid build up that results in muscles becoming tired and burning with you then stopping, so by learning how to deal with this you can then workout for longer periods of time resulting in more calories and fat being burnt off and that weight is disappearing.

This does take some time, but you at least know that whilst you are building up this resistance, your body is currently burning off fat as quickly as it needs to in order to give you energy to keep on working.

Finally, this approach results in improving the sensitivity of your body to insulin and the outcome of this is that the muscles are going to absorb the glucose, and use it to repair themselves and to get energy, rather than it being turned into fat stores. This does mean that when you burn off the fat, and then lose weight, it should stay that way rather than things fluctuating depending on how much exercise you have been doing during the week.

Using high intensity cardio to burn fat faster does indeed work, but you must be prepared to put in a lot of work in order to achieve the best possible end result. By using this approach, your body will burn off fat as it needs that sudden surge of energy and you will also build lean muscle quicker so not only will you get fitter, but you will also notice a difference when you step on those scaled and this, after all, is the important part.

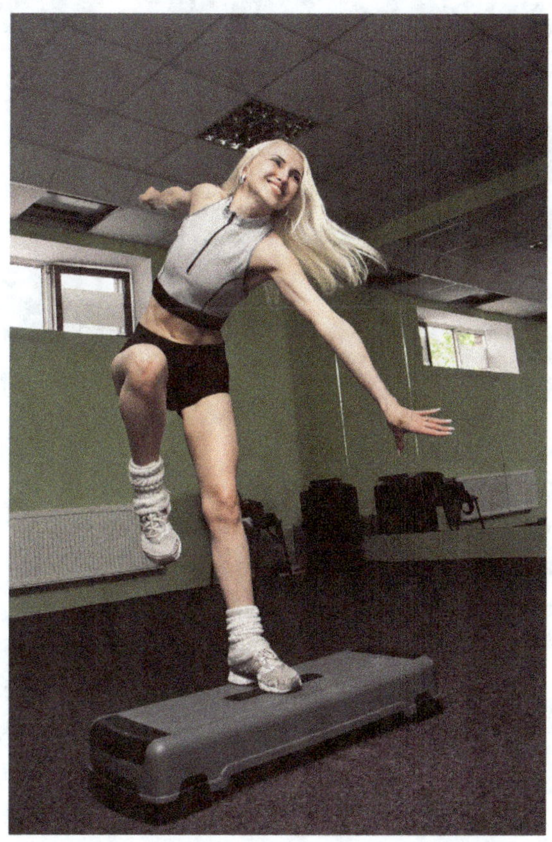

CHAPTER 6- KEY HABIT 5 – MAKE READING A HABIT

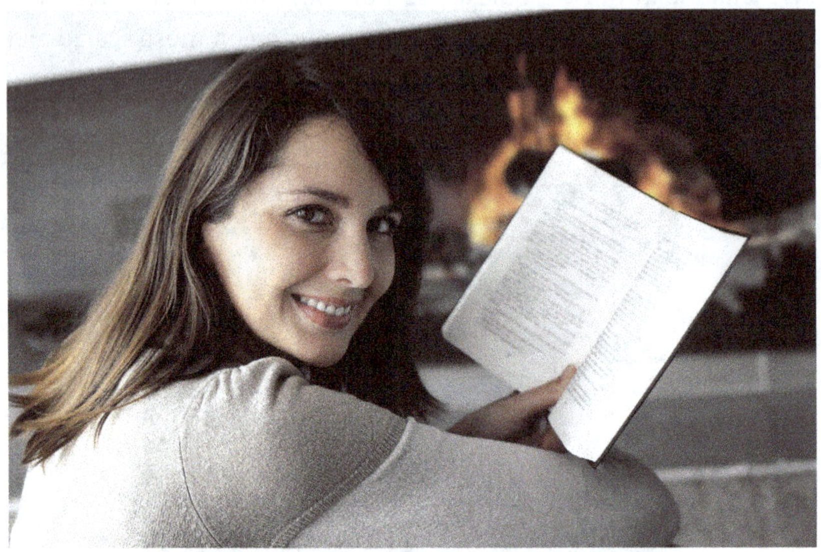

In order for you to effectively experiment in your day to day eating and still choose nutritionally excellent foods, you must understand nutrition labels on packaging. Quite often the companies that manufacture different foods will claim on the packaging that they are low fat or healthy, but the truth of the matter is that there are hidden dangers in there for people that are on different diets. Being able to read the labels can, therefore, make a huge difference in the potential success of somebody that is trying to lose weight.

First, you must look at the serving size on the label because the nutritional information that is listed on there will tend to talk about a serving size that is smaller than the overall size of the item you are looking at. This is important because a number of companies will mention a portion of say 30g and list the nutritional information for that amount, but they know most people will take double so, in actual fact, it is then nowhere near as healthy as you think.

What you need to do is to look at the serving size and then, if you eat double, you must double those figures to see how healthy it actually is.

Another key area to look at is when they discuss the percentage of the daily recommended amount that a portion covers as this can tell you a lot about what is in the product and how it can affect your diet plan.

Yet again you need to look at the serving size along with this because if the serving size is 30g and it gives you 25% of your daily recommended allowance for salt and you take 60g, then you need to double this 25% in order to get a true reflection. Do also look to see if they mention how many calories per day this recommended amount is based on as the majority will be for 2000 calories, but you may be on less than that so you must calculate it accordingly.

Finally it is worth looking at how to read the individual ingredients as they will tend to use terms such as Sodium instead of salt or they will talk about carbohydrates instead of just listing how much sugar is in it. The thinking here is that by using more professional names, then it will sound healthier and it may be an idea to look at the names on labels you have near you now and make a note of the terms used so you know if unsaturated fats are good or bad, how much vitamin B12 is good for you and that you understand what type of sugar they have put into the food and what appears in it naturally due to the ingredients.

So that is how to read nutrition labels to help lose weight and there really is nothing complex about it as long as you just take your time to read things properly. By law they must have this information printed on there, so as long as you have an understanding of the amounts of different things you should eat for your diet plan, then you should find it that bit easier to go ahead and lose that weight.

CHAPTER 7- KEY HABIT 6 – GET THAT TONED BODY

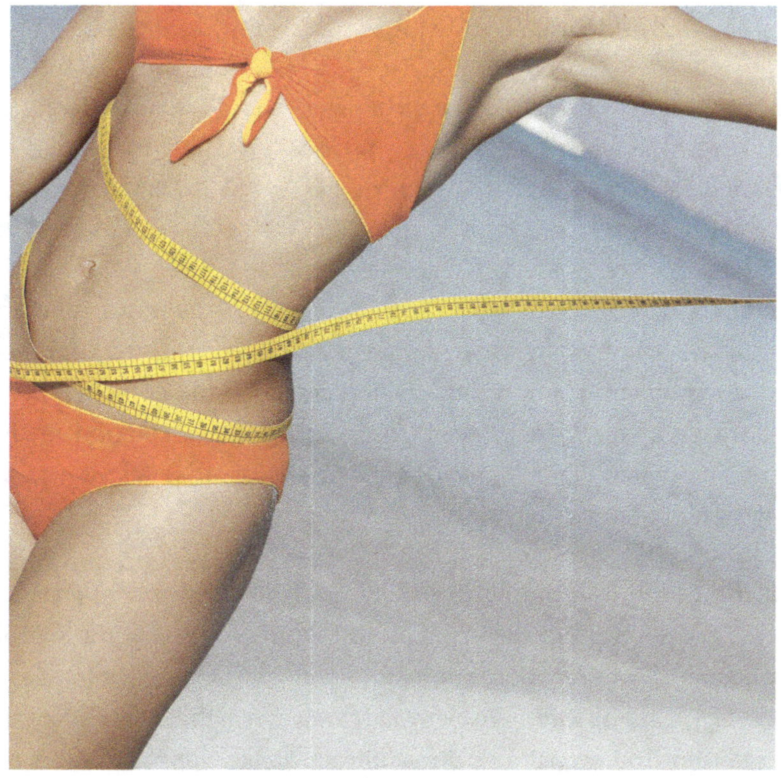

Excess weight is one of the most common problems that affect very many people from all across the globe. There is need to lose this unwanted weight so as to avoid health complications such as heart attack and other related diseases. In this chapter we will uncover resistance training exercises that can help you lose the excess fat. Examples of some of the common resistance training activities include weight lifting, sporting activities such as Basketball and Javelin, Isotonic resistance training which entails use of barbells and dumbbells. Below is a detailed guide of the importance of resistance training for losing weight.

Increase metabolic rate- The metabolic rate refers to the rate at which the body converts fats into energy for various purposes. Resistance training helps to increase the rate at which the fats are metabolized and this in turn helps to significantly reduce body fat.

Improves Body Posture- Since virtually all the physical activities in this category involves all the body muscles, they help to strengthen and increase muscles. This in turn helps one to improve body posture.

Increase Blood Circulation- For the body organs to operate optimally, they have to have sufficient and uninterrupted supply of blood rich in various nutrients such as proteins and carbohydrates. Resistance training helps to ensure that blood circulation in the body is optimal. This in turn helps to ensure that all vital body organs operate normally.

Decreases the Risk of Injuries- Losing weight involves a number of physical activities which may lead to injuries especially during the first stages. For example, new members might experience joint and muscles pains but this problem fades away as the body becomes acquainted to the activity. Resistance training will help decrease your susceptibility to injuries since the body parts will be able to withstand the pressure effectively.

Prevent cardiovascular diseases as well as Arthritis and diabetes- Excess weight has being closely linked to a number of health complications. Due to fact that these exercises will reduce and prevent accumulation of fats in the body, your chances of suffering from various cardiovascular diseases, diabetes and arthritis will be reduced significantly.

Boost Self Esteem- In most cases, persons suffering from excess weight problem are often stigmatized by the society. Fortunately, resistance training will help reduce this stigmatization and boost your self esteem.

Improves your Sleep Patterns- Excess weight can distort your sleeping pattern especially if the issue is stressing you too much. Through these physical activities, you will be able to solve this problem completely. This will in turn help you sleep much better at night as well as boost your productivity at home or at your work place.

Increase Bone Density and Strength- As the name suggest, this training will not only help you lose weight but also increase your bone density and strength. Increased bone strength will help reduce your susceptibility to injuries as well as enhance your performance of various physical tasks.

Be sure to consult a professional medical practitioner before enrolling in a particular program so as to avoid any health complications. Last but not least, ensure that your follow the instructions given by your trainer so as to achieve the full benefits from this training.

Common Misconceptions of Resistance Training

1. Women who do strength training will become bulky and muscular

This myth has been around for so many years and unfortunately a lot of women believe it. Women do not have the ability to bulk up when they do resistance training exercises to increase their metabolism. Those who bulk up are the ones that take male hormones and inject anabolic steroids into their body. These kinds of women are mostly professional body builders. Therefore if you want to achieve that bulky look, it is very clear what you have to do. However, if you just want to achieve a lean toned body, resistance training exercises will give you just that; no bulky shoulders or arms.

2. Weights and expensive gym equipment are necessary for resistance training exercises

While free weights and other gym equipment are necessary to speed up your progress, they are not necessarily the only things that you can use to build muscles. There are a variety of ways that you can build muscle and some of them include: resistance bands, bar method, Pilate's, using your own body weight and isometric training. There are many programs for resistance training that do not use any equipment yet they help people to achieve excellent results.

3. When you grow old you cannot build muscle

This is not true because studies show that even people who are 70 years old can build muscle. In addition, people who are in their 50's or even 40's can be able to build adequate muscle mass with just a few training sessions per week.

4. Resistance training requires hours and hours of training per day

This takes the crown for being the biggest misconception about resistance training that can help boost your metabolism. Experts believe that as long as you eat a healthy well balanced diet and you do not have any diseases, you will only need about 20 minutes to half an hour sessions per week for you to realize results.

It is not the hours that you spend at the gym training but it is how often you do them and how hard you push your body. It has been established that when you add even a pound of muscle, your metabolism will increase and you can burn up to a maximum of 50 calories per day.

Imagine how many calories you can burn when you add 10 pounds of muscle.

5. You will need to constantly lift heavy weights in order to maintain muscle mass

If you train every day you are likely to build more muscle and speed up your metabolism, right? Wrong! It has been proven that the people who achieve phenomenal results are the ones that take breaks in between their work out days. Muscles are built when our bodies are resting and not when they are active as most people would like to believe. The body also needs to recover after an intense work-out session.

CHAPTER 8- KEY HABIT 7 – HEALTHY PEOPLE, HEALTHY LIFESTYLE

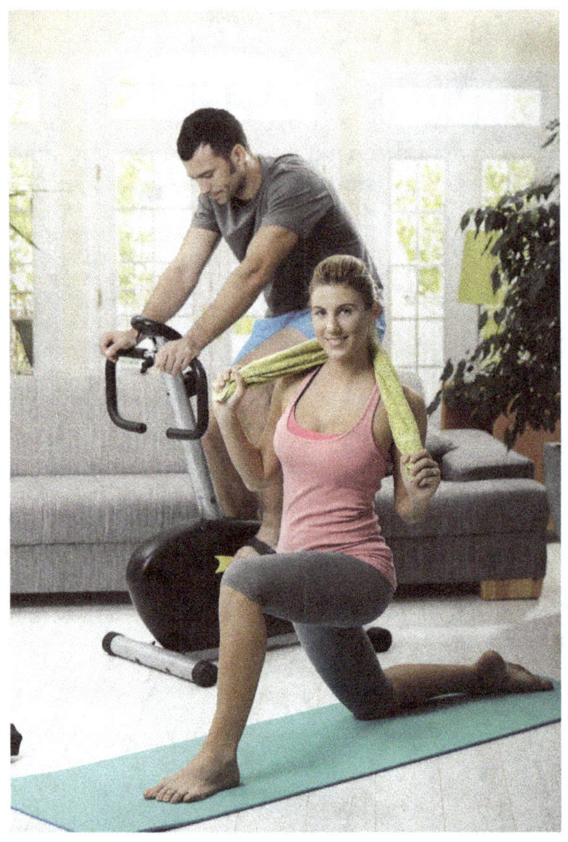

Whenever a special occasion or a holiday draws near, people often scramble for quick weight loss products or programs. While looking good in swimwear during summer is not a bad idea, looking for a short cut to weight loss can backfire. Truth is, weight loss is a lifestyle and not a fad. It is a result of a consistent effort that involves exercise, proper food intake, and the right amount of rest. This key will reveal how to achieve a healthy lifestyle that helps shed pounds permanently.

First, you have to change your perception about weight loss. It's not just a matter of watching your weight on the scale. Weight loss should be about changing your body composition by having less body fat and acquiring more muscles. For women, this means losing side handles and toning your thighs. For men, it mainly means decreasing your waist line. Lately, health experts are associating heart disease risks with a large waistline. Hence, having ripped abs is not just for aesthetic reasons but mainly for longevity. Weight loss is a goal to achieve good health; looking good should only be a consequence.

Second, you have to exercise on a daily basis if possible. Start with brisk walking if you're overweight to prevent knee injuries. Perform this activity consistently by spending at least twenty minutes a day. Or, you can try a high intensity interval training (HIIT) to jumpstart your metabolism. Samples of which are burpees, body squats, pushups, and mountain climbers. This is way shorter to perform but requires cardiovascular health and lower body weight. It shocks the body to drastically increase metabolism that results to weight loss. However, this is not advisable for people who are just beginning to exercise.

Third, educate yourself on proper food intake. People who need to lose weight should consume less than their total energy expenditure. Plus, macronutrients like protein take center stage along with complex carbohydrates. Reducing consumption of sugary food products does a lot of good to your body. Hyperlidimia, a condition where the body has high levels of cholesterol, is often triggered by obesity and diabetes.

Avoid eating fast food. Prepare meals and bring them to work. Choose lean ground meat and season them with spices. Then, make sure you have a side dish of vegetables to add more fiber in your diet.

Lastly, minimize stress in your life by managing them. Again, you can resort to exercise to shake off stress from work. Listen to relaxing music. Enjoy time with your family or pursue a hobby you love. Stress produces hormones like cortisol that sabotage our attempts at weight loss. Also, get enough sleep so your mind and body can function optimally.

As you can see, weight loss is a lifestyle and not a fad. It means prioritizing exercise over a sedentary lifestyle. It means choosing the right food to fuel your body. Most of all, it means a healthy perspective of what life is all about - taking care of yourself for your loved ones.

CHAPTER 9- ABS ROUTINE WORKOUT HABIT

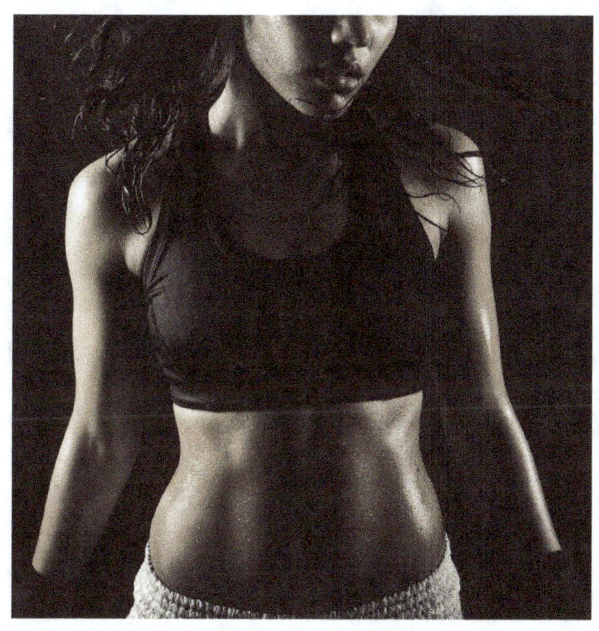

ABS ROUTINE

(MONDAY – WEDNESDAY – FRIDAY)

Exercise Order:

• Hanging leg raises (3 sets of 12 reps)

• V-Sits (3 sets of 20 reps)

• Flutter Kicks (3 sets of 1-min kicks)

• Planks (3 sets of 1-min planks)

• Side planks (4 sets of 30-second side planks on each side)

Notes:

• Do all sets for each one of these exercises in order. This abs routine isn't meant to be done like the other routines. It's meant to be done one exercise at a time (for all the sets and reps indicated) before moving on to the next exercise.

WEEKS 2 & 4: DAY 4 (Back/Biceps)

- Back -

Do 1 set of 6-12 reps performing one exercise after another. After performing all 10 exercises rest 60 seconds. Then do that series one more time.

Exercises (in this order):

• Pull Ups

• Pull Downs (wide grip)

• Bent Over Barbell Rows (wide grip)

• Bent Over Barbell Rows (close grip, hands about 6-8 inches apart)

• Reverse Grip Barbell Rows

• Bent Over Dumbbell Rows

• Reverse Grip Pull Downs

• Seated Cable Rows

• Close Grip Pull Down with V-Bar

• Straight Arm Pull Down

- Biceps -

Do 1 set of 6-12 reps. Perform all 10 exercises back-to-back with no rest between sets or exercises. Rest 60 seconds and repeat the series.

Exercises (in this order):

• Standing Barbell Curl (wide grip)

• Standing Barbell Curl Close Grip (hands spaced 8 inches apart)

• Seated Dumbbell Curl

• Incline Dumbbell Curl

• Preacher Curl with EZ curl bar (close grip)

• Preacher Curl with EZ curl bar (wide grip)

• Hammer Curls

• Reverse Grip Curls with EZ curl bar

• 1-Arm Concentration Curl

•   Standing Cable Curls

WEEKS 2 & 4: DAY 5 (Shoulders)

- Shoulders -

Do 1 set of 6-12 reps doing the 10 exercises below back-to-back without resting between sets. Rest 60 seconds and repeat the series.

Exercises (in this order):

• Seated Dumbbell Press

• Standing Dumbbell Lateral Raise

• Cable 1-Arm Lateral Raise

• Seated 1-Arm Dumbbell Lateral Raise

• Upright Rows (wide grip)

• Upright Rows (close grip)

• Bent Over Dumbbell Lateral Raise

• Bent Over Cable Lateral Raise

• Front Dumbbell Raise

• Shrugs (using a barbell)

- Abs -

Twisting Sit Ups (using a slant board if possible)

•3 x 20 reps

- Cardio –

•30 minutes

WEEKS 2 & 4: DAY 6 & 7 (Abs/Cardio)

On one of these days do 30 minutes of cardio and abs, and take the other day off. Which day you do what doesn't matter.

- Abs -

Knee Raises (use a roman chair or hanging)

•3 x 20 reps

Side Bends (or any oblique exercise)

• 3 sets (as many as you can do)

- Cardio –

• 30 minutes

NOTES FOR WEEKS 2 & 4 ROUTINES:

These "Exercise Cheat Sheets" were created so you can print them off and bring them to the gym to reference during your workouts.

They're small and condensed so you can put them in your gym bag, carry them in your pocket, or even just download the PDF of them to your phone.

Remember the main points for these workout routines:

1) For each set and exercise (excluding abs, which has its own rep scheme) you're doing 8 to 10 reps.

2) You should be using weights heavy enough that 8-10 reps bring you to failure.

3) For each muscle group on the given day, you're doing all the exercises in the series with no rest between exercises. That's one series. After you complete one full series, rest 1-2 minutes and repeat the series (so you're doing a total of 2 series for each muscle group).

4) Each group of exercises is its own "series". (Example: on Chest/Triceps days, you're doing all 6 chest exercises, resting 1-2 minutes and then doing all the chest exercises again. Then you move on to triceps, doing 2 series of those exercises. Finally, do the cardio after you're finished with those 4 series.)

5) As you progress through the series, you'll likely have to drop the weight you're using to hit the appropriate rep range as muscle fatigue will set in. You'll likely finish the series with a much lighter weight than you'd normally use, but it's going to feel heavy from

the muscle fatigue. That's expected. Don't try to overload the weights and NOT hit the rep range because you don't want to be seen using low weights. (After a month's time you'll change more physically than most other guys in the gym anyway.)

Chapter 10- Healthy People and Bodybuilders

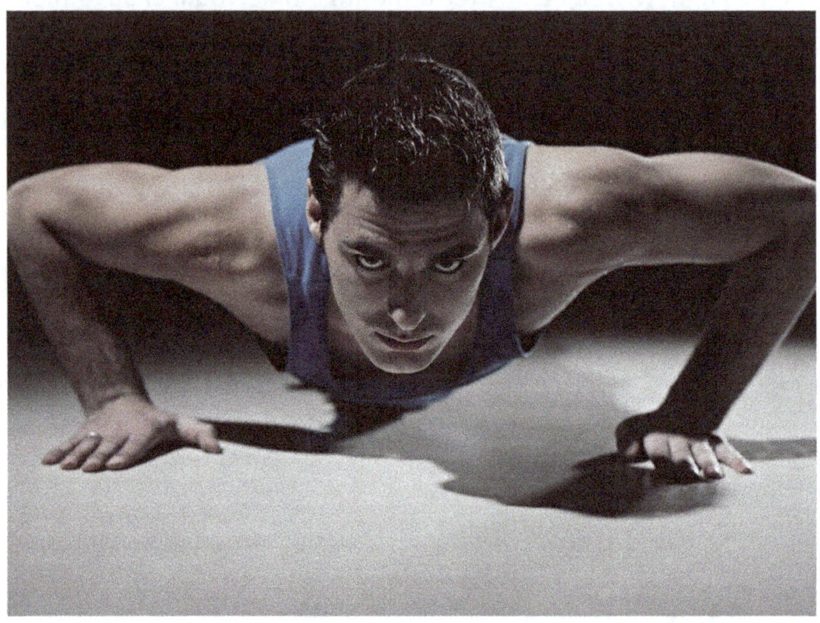

Bodybuilding is described as the process of developing your muscles by using a combination of weight training, specific caloric intake, and getting proper rest. Bodybuilding goes beyond building muscles simply to be fit, and requires more intense workouts. Some people get into "professional bodybuilding" so they can compete against others who show their physiques to a panel of judges.

People involved in competitive bodybuilding, are bodybuilders who work to develop and maintain an aesthetically pleasing (by bodybuilding standards) body and balanced physique. The bodybuilding competitors will then show off their bodies by performing a series of poses. Those involved in competitive bodybuilding will spend time practicing their pose, as this will have a big effect on how they are judged.

In competitive bodybuilding, a bodybuilder's size and shape are more important than how much he or she can lift. The sport of competitive bodybuilding should not be confused with power lifting, where they are judged on actual physical strength, or with Olympic weightlifting, where the main objective is equally split between strength and technique. Though these sports may seem superficially similar to the casual observer, each one entails a different regimen of training, diet, and basic motivation.

While exercise is certainly a key component in bodybuilding, so is nutrition. If the body doesn't get the proper nutrients to help the muscles grow, they will never reach their full potential. Since bodybuilders require high levels of muscle growth and repair, they require a specialized diet.

A bodybuilder needs more calories than the average person of the same height and weight, because it takes a higher number of calories, above their "maintenance level", in order to continue to increase muscle mass. A maintenance level of food energy, combined with cardiovascular exercise, is needed to lose body fat.

Before beginning any change in your exercise or diet routines, you should consult your doctor.

Body Building Exercise Tips

When you first begin an exercise program, regardless of whether it's weight training or cardio, your muscles immediately begin to use energy to allow them to work. For optimum health and fat burning, your bodybuilding workouts should consist of both anaerobic, and aerobic training.

Many weight training programs will tell you to do 12 repetitions of each exercise to gain muscle. The problem with that is, this approach leaves the muscles without enough tension for effective muscle gain.

High-tension, such as heavy weights, provides muscle growth, which in turn allows the muscles to grow much larger than without hightension, and also leads to a maximum gain in strength. Having longer tension time boosts the muscle size by generating the structures around the muscle fibers, which improves endurance.

The standard prescription of 8 - 12 repetitions provides a balance. But, by only using that program when you exercise, you do not generate the greater tension levels provided by the heavier weights and lesser reps, or the longer tension achieved with lighter weights and more repetitions. Change the number of reps, and adjust the weights to stimulate all types of muscle growth.

There are also those who perform the 3-Set rule, and while there's nothing wrong with the 3 sets, there is nothing amazing about it either. You see, the number of sets you perform should be based on your goals, and not on some half-century old rule. The more repetitions you do of an exercise, the fewer sets you should do, and vice versa. By using this technique, you will keep the total number of repetitions performed of an exercise equal.

Doing 3 - 4 exercises per group is also not a good idea. Here's why: Combined with 12 reps of 3 sets, the total number of reps amount to 144. If you're doing this many reps for a muscle group, you're not doing enough. Instead of doing too many different kinds of exercises, try doing 30 to 50 reps, so it should be anywhere from 2 sets of 15 reps or 5 sets of 10 reps.

Some who first start out will make the mistake of thinking the more reps you do, or the longer time you spend working on the equipment, the more muscle you build. A principal of bodybuilding says that you workout until the muscle is fatigued. Each exercise set you do is different. Depending on what your set is like, if what you do taxes the muscle, it is possible to fatigue the muscles in the first set. A good rule to follow is to create an intensity in your workout by dropping, or breaking down sets, in which you rep out or lower the weight, and continue to do reps until you either cannot do another one, or you run out of weight.

Sorting myth from truth about bodybuilding can help you design your workout, so it will be healthier and more productive. Training your mind to follow the truth about bodybuilding is like training your body. You can have discipline on two levels: body and mind.

CHAPTER 11- INCLUDE STRETCHING IN YOUR REGIMEN

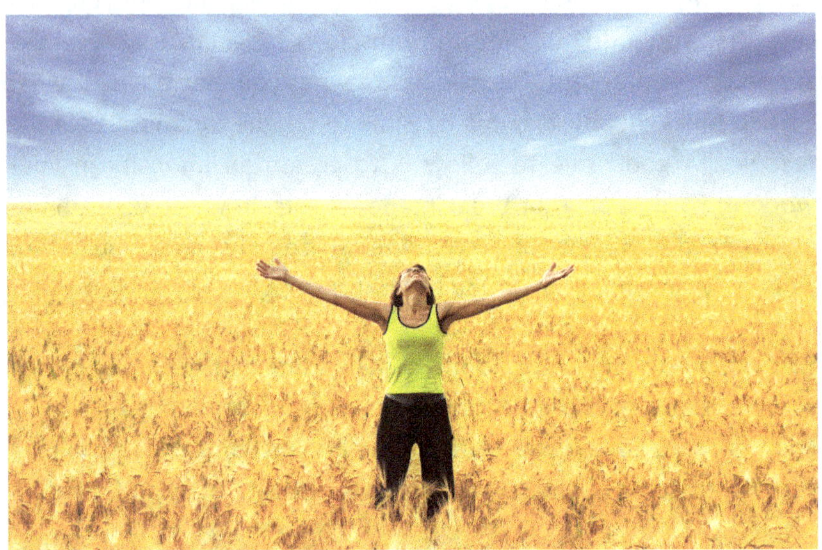

Benefits of stretching

Before beginning any exercise routine, you should do some warm-up exercises. This is usually done by performing stretching exercises, which helps prepare the body for more rigorous activity. Here are some of the benefits of stretching.

1. Gives Your Body More Range of Movement

If we are consistently doing the stretching exercises, the length of the muscles and tendons will increase. This helps expand the range of your movement. Therefore, the limbs and joints will be able to move more freely.

2. Increases Your Ability to Perform Skills

When you have a wide range of movement, you will find yourself able to do more things. For example, you can jump high without feeling any pain when you come back down on the floor.

3. Helps to Prevent Injury

By stretching, you can help prevent injury to joints, tendons and muscles. When the muscles and tendons are well flexed, they are considered to be in good working order. The muscles of the body will be able to take on more exhausting and rigorous movements, with less probability of being injured. It will also promote faster recovery from injuries (should they occur), and you'll have fewer sore muscles.

4. Helps to Reduce Muscle Tension

If you perform regular stretching exercises, it is less likely the muscles will constrict. This will definitely relieve you of any muscle pain or problems.

5. More Energy

By stretching, you'll not only be able to move more freely, you will also have more energy. Stretching will also help enhance your mood. Many people find it improves their overall confidence and well-being which makes you ready to tackle more things knowing your body is capable of handling it. The

Importance of Working Your Core Muscles

What Are Core Muscles?

Your core muscles are those muscles found in the obliques, abdominals, lower back, and the glutes areas. These 4 areas of the body are the ones that usually frame the posture of a person.

Therefore, a good posture reflects the good condition of these muscle areas.

What many people don't know is that core muscles are actually the "core" or central part for all the strength needed to carry out different physical activities. This means if an individual's core muscles are physically fit, they will maintain equilibrium of the body, and will stabilize the system every time the person is working out or moving around.

1. Strengthening Core Muscles

The main responsibility of the core muscles is to provide enough power to the body to enable it to cope with the dynamic challenges of any physical activity the person encounters.

For this reason, many health and fitness experts have realized it is relatively more important to strengthen the core muscles than the other muscles in the body. Through series of experiments and research, they have found having a stronger core can reduce your risk of many posture related health problems.

For instance, well-conditioned core muscles can project good posture.

It can also improve the endurance of the back, all the way through the day.

Why? Because the muscles included in the group of core muscles are actually the ones that initiate the proper stabilization of the whole upper and lower torso.

So, for those who desire to know and understand why it's important to strengthen the core muscles, here is a list of some of the benefits you can use as references:

This means, as you work stretching exercises into your routine, taking a particular focus on the muscles of the upper and front part of the trunk, including the abdominal and trunk muscles. By doing this, you will be strengthening the muscles of the back which extend to the spine.

2. It will help tone the muscles, thereby, avoiding further back injury

Exercising your core muscles will strengthen and tone your lower back muscles and buttocks, while stretching the hip flexors and the muscles on the front of the thighs.

When you get to this state, it will help prevent you from getting a serious lower back injury.

3. Improves physical performance

Exercising the core muscles, with slow, static stretching, is effective in relieving stiffness and enhancing flexibility. Once the flexibility has been improved, it stands to reason he will be able to perform his physical activities much more easily.

4. They do not cause sore aching muscles

Static stretching for core muscles is best for the muscles and connective tissues. Because it employs slow stretches only, it will not cause any soreness, as the quick, bouncing exercises relying on jerky muscle contractions do.

5. Lengthen muscles and avoid unbalanced footing as you get older

Core muscle exercises will lengthen the muscles that have constricted as a result of pain. It also prevents pain from vigorous exercise, if they are included at the end of each workout.

Health and fitness experts highly recommend starting a core work out immediately, and repeating the routine at least twice a week. This can be done after the workout or even during the activity, for about 10 - 20 minutes only.

Indeed, core muscles are vitally important in determining good posture. Strengthening them can absolutely eliminate those annoying back pains.

CHAPTER 12- HOW TO EFFECTIVELY PREVENT MUSCLE CRAMPS

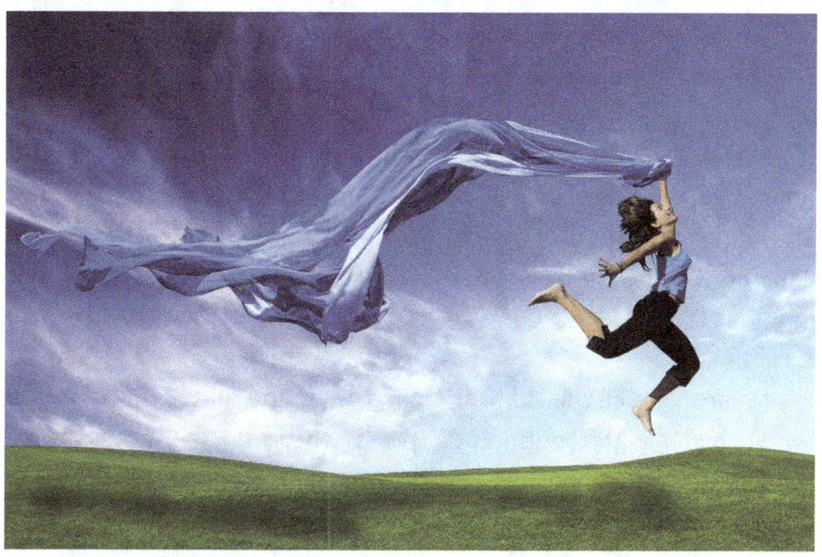

Muscle cramps are something just about everyone will experience at sometime. A muscle cramp is the involuntary tightening of a muscle, which you can usually control. They most often occur in the legs and abdomen. These cramps can put a real damper on your workout, so its best to practice healthy habits, which can help prevent muscles from cramping while you exercise.

One way to help prevent a muscle cramp is to warm up your muscles before you start your workout session. Use the mat area of the gym (or mat at home) to stretch your muscles by doing some light lifting to prepare for a more intense workout. By giving your muscles a warm up, they will expand and contract better during exercise, preventing you from getting cramps.

If you are really out of shape, you will need to warm up on a larger scale. Just remember to start off slowly, and work your way up to harder and more intense exercises. If you are an athlete just returning to your sport after the off-season or an injury, you will be more prone to muscle cramps, like those just getting started. By building on the intensity of your workouts, you will build muscle mass more quickly as well, so don't overdo it from the start, and be sure to take enough time to rest between workouts.

It's also very important to keep your muscles, and the rest of your body, hydrated. Be sure to drink lots of water before, during, and after your weight training or any other workout. You should supply your body with water before you feel thirsty, so drink at regular intervals.

If you are out in the sun, or doing anything that is making you sweat, avoid water poisoning. This is where those 'sports juices' can come in very handy. By drinking sports juices, you help to replenish all the nutrients your body is losing. If you lose too many of these nutrients, you may experience muscle spasms and cramps.

If by some chance you do get a muscle cramp, don't fret. This is normal and will most likely go away in just a few minutes, although, you may be sore a bit longer. If you get a muscle cramp, stop what you're doing, and gently stretch and massage the muscle until it is no longer cramped. If you can, apply heat, which will also help relax the muscle, and if you are sore, cold compresses will help your muscles heal.

If you continue to experience cramps regularly, or it takes a long time to get rid of them, see your doctor to make sure there is not a serious medical condition present.

Bodybuilding That Fits Your Unique Body

Everyone's body is different, so it only makes sense, not everyone should train their bodies the same way. Any professional will tell you the key to successful bodybuilding is to know your body, know your limits and know how your body will respond to certain conditions. That being said, to help optimize your bodybuilding workout, you need to determine your body type.

Everyone falls into one of 3 categories: ectomorph, mesomorph, and endomorph. By discovering the category that best fits your body, you can help find the lifestyle that will work best for you. Before engaging any lifestyle changes, you should always check with your docor.

Ectomorphs are people who naturally have little or no fat (the lucky ones). Usually, ectomorphs body types are tall and have longer limbs as well. Due to their build, most ectomorphs will choose endurance sports, like running. But, if you fall into this category, you can still become a world-class bodybuilder.

To begin, ectomorphs will need to up their calorie count and eat more throughout the day, but in smaller proportions. You should try to increase your intake by at least 500 calories per day to help put on the weight. When we say eating more, it doesn't necessarily mean eating anything you want. You will need to have a high calorie healthy diet if you want to be successful at bodybuilding.

If you are an ectomorph, you should cut most of the cardiovascular activity from your workout, and focus mainly on intense weight training. You don't want to overtrain, but you should get to the gym every 3 - 4 days for a hard full-body workout, which involves all muscle groups. It may be difficult for ectomorphs to gain muscle mass, but with a lot of hard work and dedication, it can be accomplished.

Mesomorphs are the people everyone envies. These are the people you see who eat lots of junk food, yet still have great bodies! One trap mesomorphs easily fall prey to is the mindset that because they can skip workouts or eat pizza, without any visible effect, they think it's not affecting their bodies at all. However, this is not true. Good genes may have given you a good body, but things such as heart disease will still effect you just as easily as anyone else.

Mesomorphs shouldn't need to change the amount of food they eat. But, if you fall into this category, make an effort to eat healthy foods, and lots of good carbohydrates instead of junk food. When you workout, you may choose to do a full-body training session, but it will probably be more beneficial for you to target and define muscles in specific areas.

Endomorphs also have no problem gaining muscle mass. However, unlike mesomorphs, these people also have no problem gaining weight. Diet control is the key to successful bodybuilding for endomorphs. Eat smaller meals, spread out throughout the day, and cut out the junk food.

Be sure to drink plenty of water, and try to stop eating for the day about 3 hours before you go to bed. Endomorphs shouldn't have any problem becoming muscular, but they need to hit the gym for lots of cardiovascular workouts, if possible, on a daily basis. It will help melt the fat from your body, so you can begin to see the muscles you are working to define.

Whatever your body type, bodybuilding can be the perfect sport for you. If you are sensible about your habits, and dedicated to the sport, you will find definition and muscle growth can be accomplished.

When you know the facts about bodybuilding, you can use them in your workout plan to give you a healthier and more productive workout. You can train your mind to follow the truth about bodybuilding, just as you can have discipline regarding the training of your body. Discipline on two levels; body and mind.The Difference Between Powerlifting and Bodybuilding

Its not surprising that many people think power lifting, and bodybuilding, are the same thing because many of the goals are the same. However, power lifting is actually a sport evolved from bodybuilding, and is of relatively modern origin, with the first formal competitions occurring in the mid 1960s. This sport is open to both men and women.

If you are involved in bodybuilding, you can benefit from power lifting, and vice versa. The main difference comes at the competition level. When power-lifting, your goal is to lift as much weight as possible, while in bodybuilding, your goal is to look as big and well defined as possible.

Powerlifting competitions are divided into 3 parts: the squat, the bench press, and the dead weight lift. When power lifting, the winner is determined not by how big your muscles look, but rather, how much total weight you lifted. Competitors are placed into classes determined by things such as age and experience, and are asked to lift in each of the three competitions.

Regardless whether you're a powerlifter or a bodybuilder, you'll want to eat a healthy diet. It's not enough to just eat enough calories in a day to optimize muscle building; you also need to eat the right foods. You'll want to stay away from bad carbohydrates, such as potatoes, and fried foods. Instead, your diet should include lots of pasta, green vegetables, and protein. If your body type requires it, you may need to cut back on certain foods in order to lose weight. Keep in mind though, powerlifting is not a measure of body fat or how well your muscles are defined, so packing on a few extra pounds won't effect how the judges view you. Having less body fat, though, will promote a healthier lifestyle altogether, and you will be able to feel better in the gym when you are weight training, if you cut the junk food out of your diet.

You will want to maintain a regular workout routine at the gym, just as you would if bodybuilding. While workouts are very important, it's also necessary to give your muscles some time off to rest, so they can recover and build in between workouts. You should also consider taking a full week off every 8 -12 weeks. This method is encouraged by many trainers, and has been found to be beneficial for most people because it reduces stress, allows your body to breathe, and helps you stay committed to your sport.

If you enjoy competitive sports, such as powerlifting, you can find it to be both beneficial to your health and rewarding. To get the most out of it, you should set goals for yourself before each competition, and focus on competing against your own goals instead of simply beating the other powerlifters. If you're dedicated to your diet and training and if you keep a positive attitude, you can succeed and enjoy the powerlifting world.

CHAPTER 13 BODYBUILDING IS A GOOD SPORT

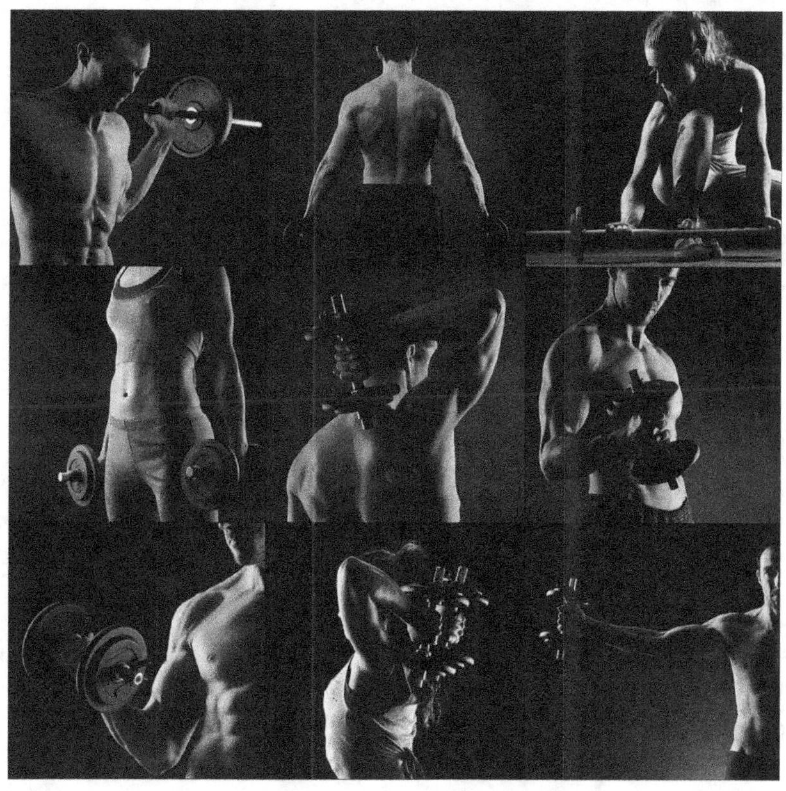

If you enjoy competitive sports, and are going to be putting a lot of time, effort, and money into building up your body, you may decide to show off your physique by participating in a bodybuilding competition.

These bodybuilding contests are held in various places all around the world and showcase some of the most physically fit bodies in the world. There are different levels of competition, so don't worry if you aren't Mr. Universe quite yet. You can still find a competition that is right for you. If you're going to get into a competitive bodybuilding contest, please be aware it will require dedication to your training, including a healthy diet and lots of exercise.

The first thing you should do, if you decide to begin competitive bodybuilding, is to find a trainer. It will be much easier to break into the competitive bodybuilding world, if you have someone with a little experience under his or her belt, to help you.

Your trainer will help you decide on a training schedule and diet plan, and also help you decide whether or not you want to take supplements. Natural training is, of course, always the best way to go, however you may want to take vitamins or other supplements to make sure your body is getting the proper nutrients it needs, even if you cut bad foods out of your diet.

The next step will be to research some of the events that may be held near you. Local events are a good place to start, if you live in a big city. If you don't live in a big city, you may have to travel some distance to find competitive bodybuilding events, so you'll need to make plans accordingly. The fees and "rules of conduct" for these events can vary, so be sure to do your homework ahead of time. Normally, you will have an orientation session the day or morning before the event, but you need to be well prepared before this, so you don't look like a novice in front of the judges.

Prior to the competition, you should not only train, but also learn how to flex while you pose, yet still look relaxed. In order to look your best, you may want to get a tan, remove body hair, and take other measures to help your body look as lean and sculpted as possible. If your trainer has participated in competitive bodybuilding, they should be able to give you advice and pointers in these areas.

After the competition, it helps to evaluate your performance, good or bad, so you can learn from your mistakes, as no one is perfect.

By learning from your past mistakes, you can perform better at future competitive bodybuilding events.

You'll want to stay focused on the staging area, and observe what the other competitors are doing that you can apply to your own performance. Once the winners have been announced, and the applause has stopped, head over to the judges' table. These judges are the experts, and they can give you a quick verbal assessment of your body, as well as some very good advice for your next competition. Don't take offense at anything negative they may tell you. Be humble, and listen to everything they have to say, both the good and bad. Before you know it, you'll be the one in the winner's circle, and it will be your turn to give advice to the new competitive bodybuilders in your area.

For some bodybuilding competitions, such as the Arnold Classic or Mr. Olympia, a competitor is only allowed to enter once he has won a qualifying amateur competition. To be qualified as a professional you may also be required to join the membership of a professional bodybuilding organization such as the IFBB.

Many natural bodybuilding organizations such as the NPA(Natural Physique Association) and NANBF (North American Natural Bodybuilding Federation) also have professional ranks.

Creatine and Bodybuilding

Creatine is a nitrogenous organic acid that naturally occurs in vertebrates, and helps supply energy to muscle cells. It is a natural substance found in some of the foods we eat, largely red meat.

In recent years, creatine has been proven to help bodybuilders in a variety of ways. Since this discovery, creatine has become one of the popular dietary supplements used by bodybuilders and powerlifters.

In the human body, creatine is synthesized mainly in the liver by the use of parts from three different amino acids - arginine, glycine, and methionine. 95% of it is later stored in the skeletal muscles, with the rest in the brain, heart, and testes.

Be sure to discuss the health risks of taking creatine supplements with your doctor, but you should be aware that there are benefits to raising your creatine levels as well.

1 When you are lifting, ATP (Adenosine 5'-triphosphate) helps your muscles contract. With each contraction, the amount of ATP in your system decreases until you are maxed out to the point where you can no longer lift. The only way to replenish ATP in your muscles is with creatine.

2 Creatine enhances your body's ability to store glycogen. Muscles use glycogen to fuel the anabolic process. Your body needs adequate glycogen to help your muscles recover after an intense workout. By doing this, your muscles grow bigger as well as faster.

3 If you aren't getting enough creatine in your diet, you may want to use a creatine supplement. Creatine is normally found in red meats, like steak. If you're a vegetarian, or someone who doesn't eat a lot of creatine-hearty foods, you may benefit from the use of supplements. Glycogen (a carbohydrate) is often achieved by what is called carb-loading (like eating lots ofpasta). By taking a creatine supplement, you will have to do less of this.

4 Creatine also increases cardiovascular activity. When you take creatine supplements, you will most likely notice the effects in your

anabolic workout, but it can also positively affect your cardiovascular exercise as well. Since creatine helps increase the amount of aerobic activity you can do before getting winded, you will be able to exercise longer and more intensely.

Although studies have shown it is generally safe to use, creatine is not for everyone. Unlike a lot of anabolic steroids and other supplements on the market, you should not start using creatine without first consulting with a doctor. You also want to be sure you are using creatine in the right amounts. Although the label should give you a general idea on how to use it, to use it most efficiently you should calculate the amount you want to use in accordance with your weight and percentage of body fat. The result of increased creatine in the body is the chemical creatinine, which is normally easily flushed out of the body through the kidneys. If you have kidney problems, however, increased amounts of creatinine can be harmful to your health. As with any substance, you must use common sense when taking creatine. If you don't abuse the use of creatine, it can help you achieve results faster.

The Down Side of Supplements

Many people take dietary supplements to help them stay healthy, but many bodybuilders abuse supplements, in an effort to get bigger muscles faster. The most commonly abused drug among bodybuilders is the anabolic steroid. While its true you may see results in less time than a natural bodybuilder, the disadvantages of using steroids greatly outweigh the benefits.

The first thing you should know about steroids, is they are illegal. You also need to know that competitive bodybuilders often have to undergo drug tests before they will be allowed to enter an event. If you get caught with steroids, it can ruin your reputation both in and out of the bodybuilding world. The negative side effects of steroids are not only the legal aspects. Using steroids can do some serious damage to your body, as well as your overall health.

Even though men and women may react differently to steroids, they both face the same types of dangers. For example, steroids will cause a man's testicles to shrink, sperm count to drop, have a deeper voice, hair loss, and make him develop breasts. Women too will experience deepened voices and hair loss, as well as enlargement of the clitoris, and increased growth of facial hair. In teenagers, who have not yet finished growing, it will stunt their growth. If these side effects haven't put a scare into you yet, continue reading. It can get much worse.

For one thing, steroids can damage your liver by causing you to develop jaundice; a disease with flu-like symptoms that turns your skin yellow. Steroids have also been known to cause cancer and liver tumors. Perhaps the worst side effect is the one that affects the heart.

Using steroids can cause enlargement of the heart, as well as hardening of the arteries, both health issues are precursors to heart disease, and in the end heart failure.

People who abuse these supplements have also been known to develop skin spots, acne, trembling, and uncontrollable anger that makes user become physically violent.

Truth be told, steroids are only useful if you are a dedicated bodybuilder already, so you won't gain any muscle mass simply by popping pills or injecting yourself. Steroids help your muscles recover from training, so while most body builders need at least 48 hours between sessions to see results, users are ready to train again in a few hours. Therefore, users can build muscles faster.

You must keep in mind, just because things happen faster, does not always mean its better. There are some bodybuilders who are pushing for steroids to be legal when used responsibly, but professionals generally agree that abusing steroids will result in an untimely death.

It is not necessary to use steroids to achieve the kind of body, bodybuilders admire. Healthy professional bodybuilders state that there are good training principals, which include the importance of having a nutrient-rich diet, along with the proper rest. Having both nutrition and rest will create a body others will envy.

CHAPTER 14- FACTS ABOUT BODY BUILDING

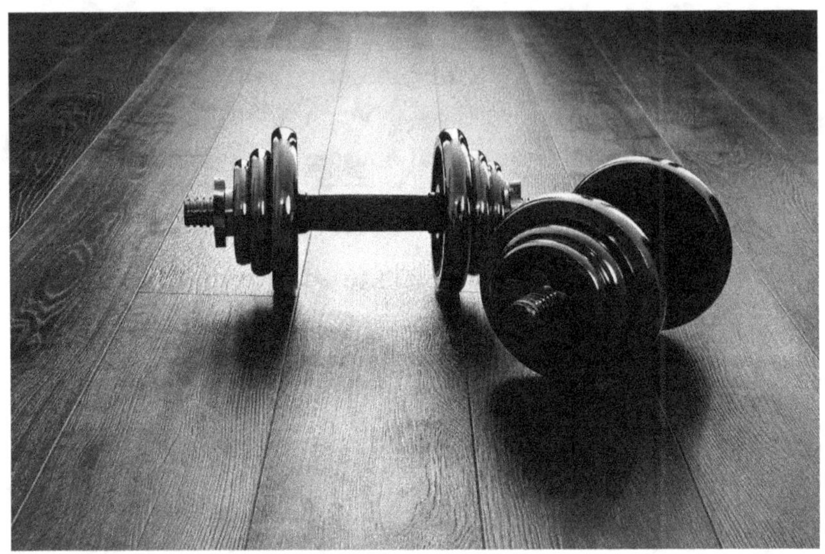

Bodybuilding attracts enthusiasts for many reasons. One of the more popular reasons among us is that they love to build those big muscles to impress the girls. Bodybuilding is also a popular way to lose weight because when you build muscle you increase your metabolism. Metabolism helps to burn calories and then you lose weight. There are those who do bodybuilding as a career because they enjoy the competitions, intense training and thrill of success. What ever your reason for bodybuilding, there are important aspects of the art that you should keep in mind to be successful. There are plenty of myths surrounding bodybuilding and sorting truth from myth will help you to be successful.

Understanding proper diet can aid you in bodybuilding. Many people make the mistake of thinking that all foods containing fat are bad for your body when bodybuilding. The real truth is that a proper balance of fat and other food groups can accelerate your physical development. It can also be underestimated concerning how important protein is to the bodybuilder. On average a bodybuilder should consume 1.2 g of protein per lb. of bodyweight. Protein is not the only important nutritional component of bodybuilding, achieving the adequate ratio of carbohydrate to protein consumption is also important.

It is not necessary to use steroids to achieve the kind of body, bodybuilders admire. Healthy professional bodybuilders state that there are good training principals that include the importance of having a nutrient-rich diet along with the proper rest. Having both nutrition and rest will create the body that others will envy.

It is also a misconception that those who start bodybuilding may have and that is that they should work faster or do more reps to build muscle. The truth is that you need to rest and workout for best results. A good schedule is to alternate workout days with rest days. Another good idea is to build your rep sequence by 5. This workout/rest and rep build up by 5 is a good combination to keep in mind to build muscle mass.

Some who first start out will make the mistake in thinking that the more reps you do or the longer time you spend working on the equipment, the more muscle you build. A principal of bodybuilding says that you workout until the muscle is fatigued. Each exercise set you do is different. Depending on what your set is like, it is possible to fatigue out in the first set, if what you do taxes out the muscle. A good rule to follow is to create an intensity in your workout by dropping or break-down sets in which you rep out or lower the weight and then continue to do reps until you either cannot do another rep or you run out of weight.

When you know the true facts about bodybuilding you can use them in your workout plan to give you a healthier and more productive workout. You can train your mind to follow the truth about bodybuilding much like you can have the discipline regarding the training of your body. Discipline on two levels - body and mind.

CHAPTER 15- THE DISCIPLINED ART OF BODYBUILDING

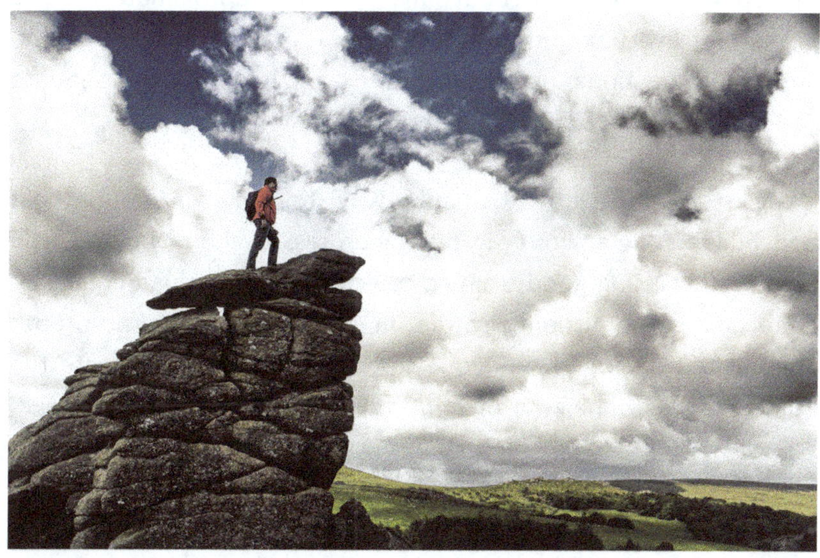

People are interested in bodybuilding for many reasons. The popular one among guys is so to build muscle and look good for the gals. Bodybuilding is popular among those who want to lose weight because building muscle increases your metabolism, which helps you to burn more calories needed to take off extra pounds. Bodybuilding can also be a career for those who love competition, intense training and the thrill of accomplishment. No matter why you decide to join the art of bodybuilding, there are some important aspects of the art that you should keep in mind. It is easy to confuse myth with reality and as with any art form that requires discipline, knowing the true facts can help to keep you on the right track towards success.

Proper diet is very important when it comes to sculpting your body. Many people mistakenly think that all fat containing foods are bad and avoid them all together. The truth is that it actually is good to include the proper fats in the right ratio to other food groups to enhance your physical development. Most people underestimate the importance of protein needed by the body when taking part in this sport. The average bodybuilder needs approximately 1.2 g protein for every pound of bodyweight. Protein is only one of the important nutritional needs of muscle growth, achieving adequate carbohydrate/protein ratio in your diet is also important.

Using steroids is not the only way to get the body most bodybuilders are envious of. Healthy professional bodybuilders will tell you that using good training principals and understanding the importance of a nutrient-rich diet in combination with the proper amount of rest will give anyone the edge you need to create the body that will be the envy of your family and friends.

Another misconception especially for those just are just starting out in bodybuilding is that the more you work out the faster you will build muscle. The truth is that you need to rest in between your workout days for optimum results. You need to do an alternate schedule like: workout day, rest day, workout day, rest day. You also will want to build your rep sequence by 5. This combination of workout/rest and increasing the rep sequence will give you the muscle mass that you desire.

Many who start out will mistakenly think that the more reps you complete or the longer time you spend on the equipment or lifting bells the more muscle you will build. One of the principals of bodybuilding is that you work out until the muscle is fatigued. Each exercise set is different. Depending on what you are doing, you can fatigue out muscle fibers in just one set, if what you are doing completely taxes out the muscle. A good rule of thumb is to create a kind of intensity in your workout where you drop or break-down sets in which you can actually rep out, by lowering the weight and then continuing doing reps until you either cannot do another rep or you run out of weight.

Knowing the true facts about bodybuilding and incorporating them into your workout plan will give you a healthier, more productive workout. Train your mind to stick to the truth about bodybuilding so that your workout discipline will play out on two levels, your body and your mind.

Chapter 16- Good Tip on How to Do Bodybuilding Successfully

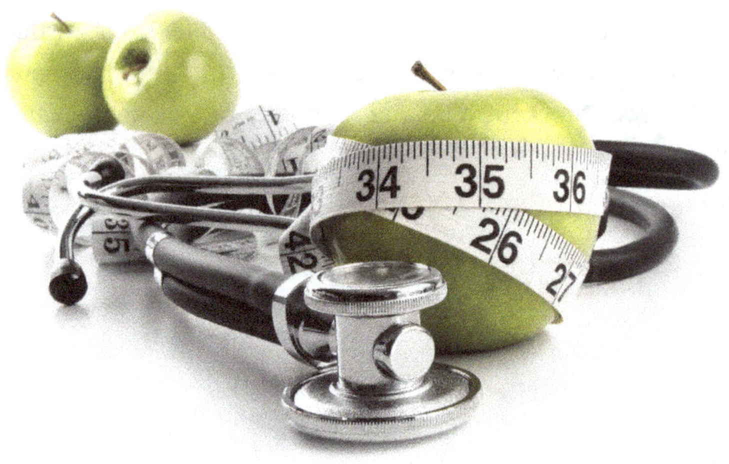

There are many reasons why people are attracted to bodybuilding. One of the most popular reasons is that guys like to build big muscles to impress the girls. Bodybuilding is also popular among those who want to lose weight. The reason bodybuilding is good for losing weight is that building muscle increases your metabolism. Increased metabolism helps to burn calories which in turns takes the weight off. Some use bodybuilding as a career choice because they love the competitions, intense training and the excitement of the sport. No matter what your reason is for bodybuilding, there are some important things to keep in mind while doing it. It is easy to become confused about what you hear or read concerning bodybuilding as there are many myths floating around. Knowing truth from myth can help you to make good decisions regarding your workouts that will lead to bodybuilding success.

Proper diet is very important when it comes to sculpting your body. Many people mistakenly think that all fat containing foods are bad and avoid them all together. The truth is that it actually is good to include the proper fats in the right ratio to other food groups to enhance your physical development. Most people underestimate the importance of protein needed by the body when taking part in this sport. The average bodybuilder needs approximately 1.2 g protein for every pound of bodyweight. Protein is only one of the important nutritional needs of muscle growth, achieving adequate carbohydrate/protein ratio in your diet is also important.

Steroids are not the only way to get the body desired by bodybuilders. Those professionals who value being healthy will tell you that good training principals include the understanding that you need to combine a nutrient-rich diet with the proper amount of rest. This proper combo will give your the edge you need to create the body that family and friends will envy.

^^Another misconception especially for those just are just starting out in bodybuilding is that the more you work out the faster you will build muscle. The truth is that you need to rest in between your workout days for optimum results. You need to do an alternate schedule like: workout day, rest day, workout day, rest day. You also will want to build your rep sequence by 5. This combination of workout/rest and increasing the rep sequence will give you the muscle mass that you desire.

Many beginners to bodybuilding will make the mistake of thinking that more reps you complete or the more equipment time or dumbbell time you log in, the faster you build muscle. A principal of bodybuilding is that it is important to workout until the muscle is fatigued. Each set is different and depending on what exercise you are doing, you may actually fatigue out muscle fibers in one set.

You should concentrate on creating the kind of intensity in your workout that will allow you to drop or break-down sets so that you can actually rep out, by lowering the weight and then continue reps until you either cannot complete another rep or you run out of weight.

Knowing the true facts about bodybuilding and incorporating them into your workout plan will give you a healthier, more productive workout. Train your mind to stick to the truth about bodybuilding so that your workout discipline will play out on two levels, your body and your mind.

Chapter 17- Myths and Truths Surrounding Bodybuilding

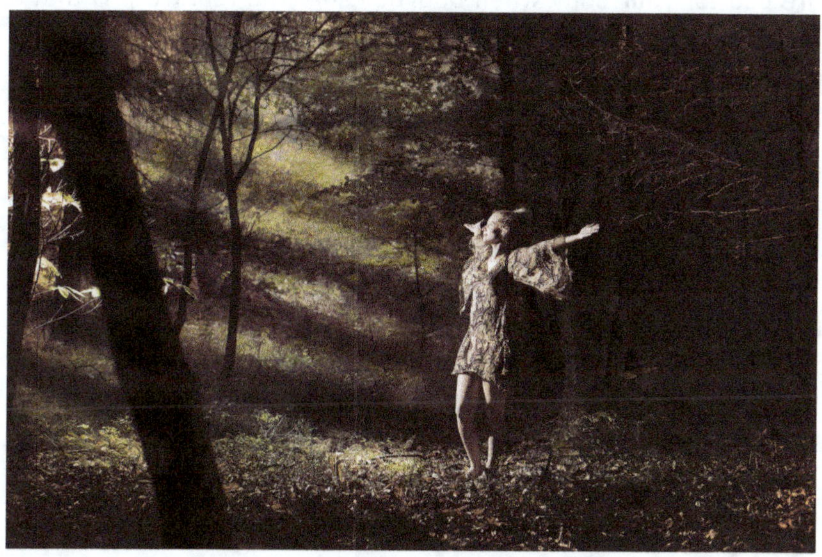

There are many reasons why people are attracted to bodybuilding. One of the most popular reasons is that guys like to build big muscles to impress the girls. Bodybuilding is also popular among those who want to lose weight. The reason bodybuilding is good for losing weight is that building muscle increases your metabolism. Increased metabolism helps to burn calories which in turns takes the weight off.

Some use bodybuilding as a career choice because they love the competitions, intense training and the excitement of the sport. No matter what your reason is for bodybuilding, there are some important things to keep in mind while doing it. It is easy to become confused about what you hear or read concerning bodybuilding as there are many myths floating around. Knowing truth from myth can help you to make good decisions regarding your workouts that will lead to bodybuilding success.

Understanding proper diet can aid you in bodybuilding. Many people make the mistake of thinking that all foods containing fat are bad for your body when bodybuilding. The real truth is that a proper balance of fat and other food groups can accelerate your physical development. It can also be underestimated concerning how important protein is to the bodybuilder. On average a bodybuilder should consume 1.2 g of protein per lb. of bodyweight. Protein is not the only important nutritional component of bodybuilding, achieving the adequate ratio of carbohydrate to protein consumption is also important.

Steroids are not the only way to get the body desired by bodybuilders. Those professionals who value being healthy will tell you that good training principals include the understanding that you need to combine a nutrient-rich diet with the proper amount of rest. This proper combo will give your the edge you need to create the body that family and friends will envy.

It is also a misconception that those who start bodybuilding may have and that is that they should work faster or do more reps to build muscle. The truth is that you need to rest and workout for best results. A good schedule is to alternate workout days with rest days. Another good idea is to build your rep sequence by 5. This workout/rest and rep build up by 5 is a good combination to keep in mind to build muscle mass.

Many beginners to bodybuilding will make the mistake of thinking that more reps you complete or the more equipment time or dumbbell time you log in, the faster you build muscle. A principal of bodybuilding is that it is important to workout until the muscle is fatigued. Each set is different and depending on what exercise you are doing, you may actually fatigue out muscle fibers in one set. You should concentrate on creating the kind of intensity in your workout that will allow you to drop or break-down sets so that you can actually rep out, by lowering the weight and then continue reps until you either cannot complete another rep or you run out of weight.

When you know the true facts about bodybuilding you can use them in your workout plan to give you a healthier and more productive workout. You can train your mind to follow the truth about bodybuilding much like you can have the discipline regarding the training of your body. Discipline on two levels - body and mind.

Chapter 18- Reasons Why People Likes Bodybuilding

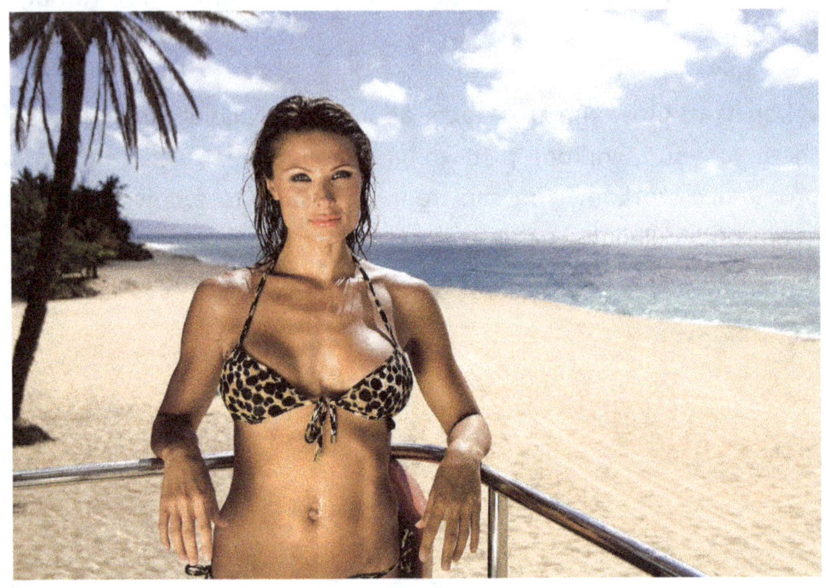

There are many reasons why people are attracted to bodybuilding. One of the most popular reasons is that guys like to build big muscles to impress the girls. Bodybuilding is also popular among those who want to lose weight. The reason bodybuilding is good for losing weight is that building muscle increases your metabolism. Increased metabolism helps to burn calories which in turns takes the weight off.

Some use bodybuilding as a career choice because they love the competitions, intense training and the excitement of the sport. No matter what your reason is for bodybuilding, there are some important things to keep in mind while doing it. It is easy to become confused about what you hear or read concerning bodybuilding as there are many myths floating around. Knowing truth from myth can help you to make good decisions regarding your workouts that will lead to bodybuilding success.

You cannot skimp on the importance of proper diet when it comes to bodybuilding. The myth in the minds of most people is that fat is bad. The truth is that not all fat is bad, it is actually healthy to have a proper ratio of fats to other food groups for a well rounded physical development. Protein has a very important role in bodybuilding. On average, a bodybuilder needs 1.2 g of protein for every pound of bodyweight. Protein is just one of the important nutrient needs for the muscle growth desired by those participating in this sport. It is important to maintain a proper carbohydrate/protein ratio in your diet.

Steroids are not the only way to get the body desired by bodybuilders. Those professionals who value being healthy will tell you that good training principals include the understanding that you need to combine a nutrient-rich diet with the proper amount of rest. This proper combo will give your the edge you need to create the body that family and friends will envy.

Another myth is that working fast or for long periods will get the body you desire. The truth is that you will get your results quicker by alternating workout days with rest days. You can also increase your rep sequence by 5 in combination with the workout/rest sequence to build the muscle mass you desire.

Many beginners to bodybuilding will make the mistake of thinking that more reps you complete or the more equipment time or dumbbell time you log in, the faster you build muscle. A principal of bodybuilding is that it is important to work out until the muscle is fatigued. Each set is different and depending on what exercise you are doing, you may actually fatigue out muscle fibers in one set. You should concentrate on creating the kind of intensity in your workout that will allow you to drop or break-down sets so that you can actually rep out, by lowering the weight and then continue reps until you either cannot complete another rep or you run out of weight.

Sorting myth from truth about bodybuilding can help you in designing your workout so that you will have a healthier more productive workout. Training your mind to follow the truth about bodybuilding is like training your body. You can have discipline on two levels body and mind.

CONCLUSION

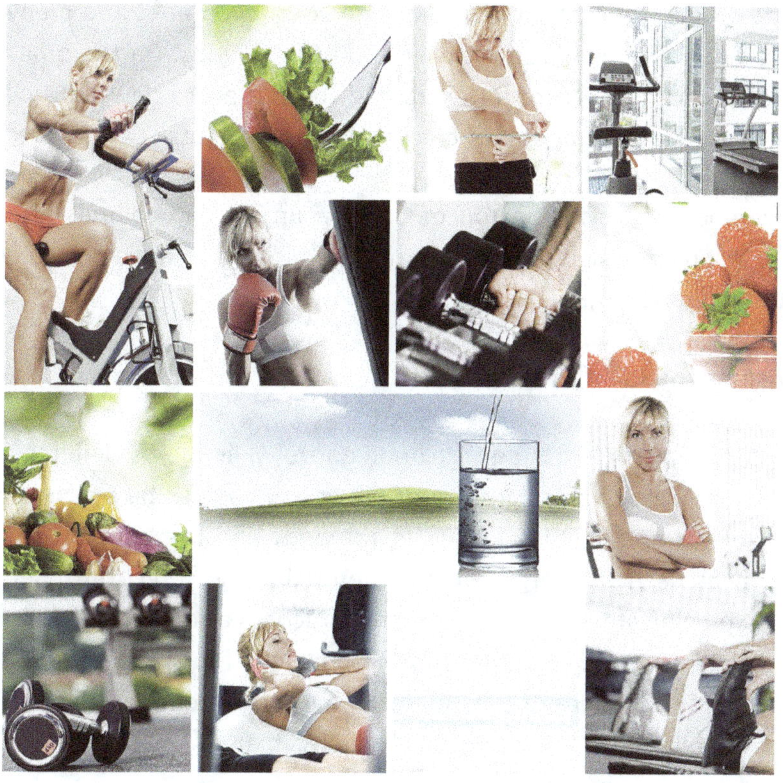

As we close out this guide, we will cover a few extra tips and tricks that will help tremendously in transforming your body. Some tips might require you to adjust your lifestyle entirely. However, they are of great assistance in losing weight.

Exercise

It's the surest and most natural way to lose weight. Exercising can be done in so many ways to fit into your daily activities. For instance, you can decide to cycle to and from your work place or shopping center instead of taking a bus. On the other hand, you can opt to use the stairs instead of the elevator. Other activities like walking, jogging and running will also contribute to weight loss.

You can make exercising fun too, like playing basket ball with your peers or kids, going on long walks with your loved ones and many more fun activities that eventually will burn calories. On the other hand, you can structure an exercising routine every day that will involve at least 30 minutes of cardiovascular exercises.

Remember, exercises on top of burning up fat and calories also help in building a lean muscles mass which is essential for the body's metabolic rate.

Consume the Right Drinks

If it's not possible to quit alcohol entirely, limit yourself to a maximum of two on isolated cases when you have to take alcohol. Alcohol has no nutritional value to the body and the body usually uses it as its first energy source. Eventually, the food consumed ends up being stored as fat in the body. Alcohol also influences you to eat the wrong type of foods, preferably junk foods that are high in calories. It's, therefore, essential to avoid alcohol consumption, or to limit its consumption, as much as possible.

Similarly, avoid fruit drinks and soda. Instead opt for diet drinks and plenty of water. Water suppresses the regular urges to eat and consequently help you lose some weight. It also keeps the body hydrated, which is ideal for nutrients' release to the body.

Green tea is also favorite beverage for people on a weight loss program. Studies have demonstrated that consuming green tea leads to more calories being burnt faster than those who do not consume it.

Consume the Right Foods

Eat the right foods that will not contribute to weight gain but rather to weight loss. Grape fruit has been found effective in helping people lose weight. Consuming half a grape fruit three times a day burns more calories by boosting the body's metabolism. On the other hand, avoid or minimize on the consumption of fats, especially animal fats as they are high in cholesterol. Opt for skim milk and low fat cheese. Similarly, consume lean meat, preferably white meat. In addition, opt for unprocessed foods as their calories and fat content is lower. On the other hand, if you have to consume processed food, like bread, opt for the whole grain bread as its high in dietary fiber content. Fiber assists in burning calories.

Also things to avoid are, refined sugar containing products and junk food. Look for sugar substitutes to use in the place of sugar. Junk food is low in nutritional value and high in calories content. Avoid it as well. However, ensure you consume plenty of fruits and vegetables and minimize on starch products for an almost ideal body weight.

About the Author

Walter Gregory is born and raised in Sacramento, California. He is a fitness and health enthusiast who is more than willing to share his experiences and knowledge about being healthy and having a healthy living. He believes that this book should guide other people to achieve a happier and longer life.

Before leading a healthy lifestyle, he was once an overweight teenager who was suffering from low self-esteem due to his physical appearance.